Understanding The Sirtfood Diet

The Succinct Guide Lose Weight By Activating Your Skinny Gene With Easy Recipes And A Sirtfood Meal Plan To Help You Get Started

Serena Baxter

© Copyright 2021 - All rights reserved.

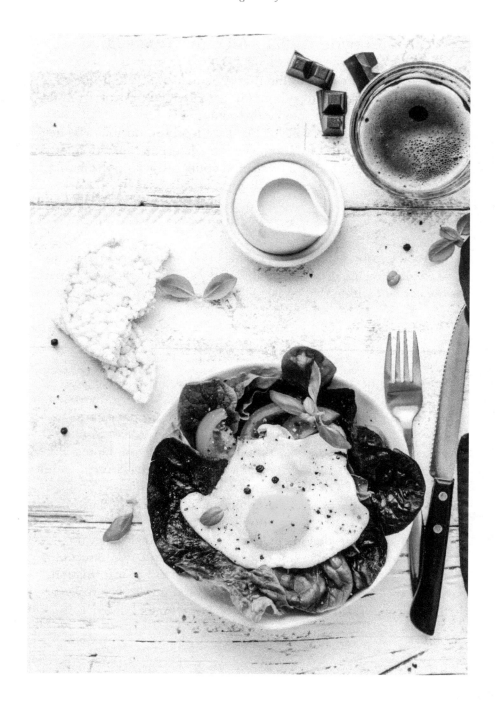

TABLE OF CONTENTS

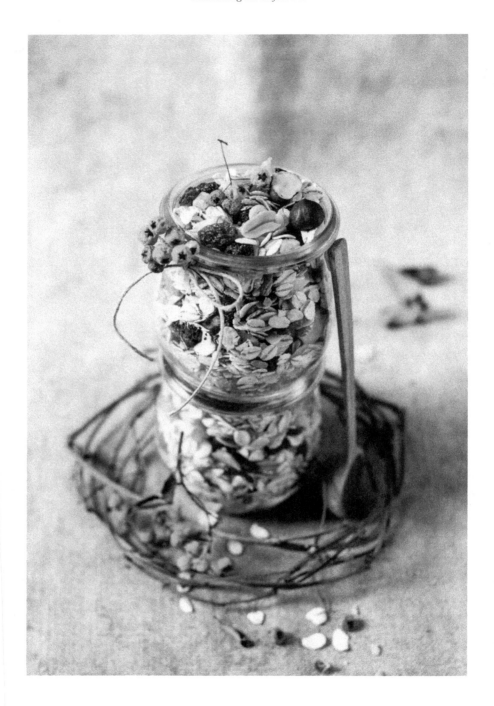

INTRODUCTION

The official Sirtfood Diet combines a short calorie restriction phase with a long-term commitment to nutrient-dense sirtuin-activating foods.

How you eat is your diet; restricting how you eat is dieting. Aside from the first week, Stage 1, the Sirtfood diet is not a traditional diet in that, instead of merely restricting calories, you focus on increasing nutrition and improving quality.

There are only 2 stages in the Sirtfood Diet, which take up 3 weeks of your life. Still, those 3 weeks are designed to set the stage for incorporating sirtfoods into your lifelong diet, eliminating your need to ever resort to dieting again.

The average American consumes many solid fats and sugars, refined grains, sodium, and saturated fat. They also under-consume vegetables, fruits, whole grains, and the nationally recommended intake of dairy and oils.

If this sounds like it matches your current eating patterns, don't be too hard on yourself, you're certainly not alone. And you've been practically brainwashed into adopting these poor nutrition habits. The number of fast-food restaurants continues to grow, as do your options for pre-made, packaged foods full of empty calories, and misleading promises. When you live on a diet of these foods devoid of all nutrition for too long, you find yourself getting sick and overweight. So, you turn to the industry that profits off of your poor health, the diet industry.

Sirtfood Diet is the newest approach to fast weight loss without extreme diet by stimulating the same 'skinny gene' mechanisms, typically just through fasting and exercise. Other foods varieties contain chemical substances known as polyphenols that stress our cells lightly, allowing genes to replicate the effects of fasting and exercise. The Sirtuin pathways, which affect metabolism, age, and mood, are guided by the food rich in polyphenols, like broccoli, dark chocolate, and red wine. However, a diet sufficient in these Sirtfoods starts to lose weight without sacrificing muscle while maintaining excellent health.

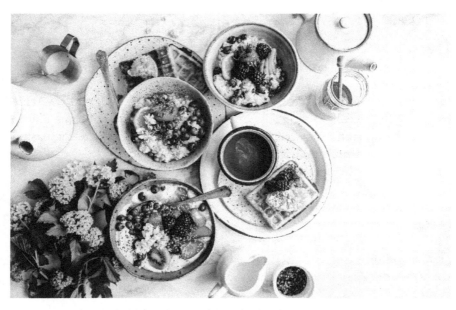

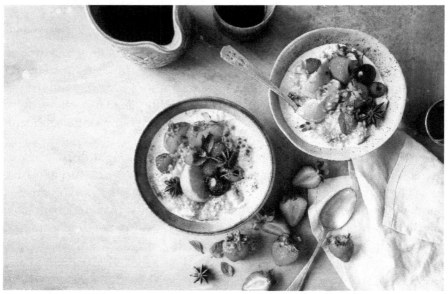

APPETIZER AND SNACK RECIPES

1. <u>Raw Vegan Coffee Cashew Cream Cake</u>

Preparation Time: 12 minutes Cooking Time: 37 minutes

Servings: 4

Ingredients:

- Coffee cashew cream

- 2 cups raw cashews

- 1 tsp of ground vanilla bean

- 3 tbsp. melted coconut oil

- ¼ cup raw honey

- 1/3 cup very strong coffee or triple espresso shot

Directions:

1. Blend all ingredients for the cream, pour it onto the crust and refrigerate.

2. Garnish with coffee beans.

Nutrition: 153 Calories 1g Fat 2g Protein

2. <u>Blackberry Peach Compote</u>

Preparation Time: 8 minutes

Cooking Time: 24 minutes

Servings: 12

Ingredients:

- ¼ cup Sauvignon Blanc wine

- 2 Tbsps. Xylitol

- 1 tsp ground ginger

- 1 tsp Cinnamon

- 3 medium peaches

- ¼ cup blackberries

- ½ tsp thick it up

Directions:

1. In a large saucepan, combine the wine, Xylitol, ginger, peaches, and cinnamon.

2. Simmer for 15 minutes.

3. Add the blackberries. Simmer another 5 minutes, until berries are tender.

4. Stir in the thick it up. Simmer approximately 5 minutes.

5. Remove from heat. Cool to room temperature. Serve.

Nutrition: 35 Calories 0.2g Fat 0.5g Protein

3. <u>Sirt Energy Balls</u>

Preparation Time: 9 minutes

Cooking Time: 11 minutes

Servings: 5

Ingredients:

- 1 cup old fashion ginger, dried

- 1/4 cup quinoa cooked

- 1/4 cup shredded unsweetened coconut

- 1/3 cup dried cranberry/raisin blend

- 1/3 cup dark chocolate chips

- 1/4 cup slivered almonds

- 1 Tbsp reduced-fat peanut butter

Directions:

1. Cook quinoa in orange juice. Boil and simmer for 4 minutes. Let cool. Combine chilled quinoa and the remaining ingredients into a bowl.

2. With wet hands and combine ingredients and roll in golden ball sized chunks.

3. Set at a Tupperware and chill until the firm.

Nutrition: 80 Calories 7g Fat 2.5g Protein

4. <u>Celery and Raisins Snack Salad</u>

Preparation Time: 16 minutes Cooking Time: 0 minutes

Servings: 4

Ingredients:

- ½ cup raisins

- 4 cups celery, sliced

- ¼ cup parsley, chopped

- ½ cup walnuts, chopped

- Juice of ½ lemon

- 2 tbsp. extra virgin olive oil

- Salt and black pepper to the taste

Directions:

1. In a salad bowl, mix celery with raisins, walnuts, parsley, lemon juice, oil, and black pepper, toss, divide into small cups and serve as a snack.

Nutrition: 120 Calories 1g Fat 5g Protein

5. <u>Yogurt & Fruit Jam Parfait</u>

Preparation Time: 6 minutes

Cooking Time: 5 minutes

Servings: 6

Ingredients:

- 3 cups Mixed Berries

- 1 tbsp. Lemon Juice

- 7/8 cup Honey

- 2 tsp. Fruit Pectin

- 1 cup Granola

- 3 cups Greek Yoghurt

Directions:

1. For making this healthy jam, you need to place the mixed berries, honey, lemon juice, and pectin in the blender pitcher.

2. Next, pulse the mixture 3 to 4 times and then press the 'sauce/ dip' button.

3. Now, transfer the jam to a safe heat container and then place it in the refrigerator for 2 to 3 hours.

4. Once the jam is chilled, layer 1/3 cup of the Greek Yoghurt into the bottom of the parfait glass.

5. After that, spoon in a jam into it and then add the granola.

6. Serve immediately.

Nutrition: 154 calories 4g fat9g protein

BREAKFAST RECIPES

6. Spiced Scrambled Eggs

Preparation Time: 13 minutes

Cooking Time: 4 minutes

Servings: 2

Ingredients:

- 2 teaspoon extra virgin olive oil

- 1/4 cup (40g) red onion, finely chopped

- 1/2 bell pepper, finely chopped

- 6 medium eggs

- 1/2 cup (100ml) milk

- 1 teaspoon ground turmeric

- 4 tablespoons (10g) parsley, finely chopped

Direction

1. Pre-heat oil in a frying pan and cook red onion and bell pepper until soft but not browned.

2. Whisk the eggs, milk, turmeric, and parsley. Add to the hot pan and continue cooking over low to medium heat, constantly moving the egg mixture around the pan to scramble it and stop it from sticking/burning.

3. When you have achieved your desired consistency, serve.

Nutrition 143 Calories 11g Fat 8g Protein

7. <u>Mushroom Scramble Eggs</u>

Preparation Time: 11 minutes

Cooking Time: 6 minutes

Serving: 2

Ingredients

- 2 tbsp

- 1 teaspoon ground garlic

- 1 teaspoon mild curry powder

- 20g lettuce, approximately sliced

- 1 teaspoon extra virgin olive oil

- 1/2 bird's eye peeled, thinly chopped

- a couple of mushrooms, finely chopped

- 5g parsley, finely chopped

Direction

1. Mix the curry and garlic powder and then add just a little water till you've achieved a light glue.

2. Steam the lettuce for two -- 3 minutes.

3. Heat the oil in a skillet over a moderate heat and fry the chili and mushrooms 2-- three minutes till they've begun to soften and brown.

4. Insert the eggs and spice paste and cook over moderate heat, then add the carrot and then proceed to cook over a moderate heat for a further minute. In the end, put in the parsley, mix well, and function.

Nutrition 148 Calories 7g Fat 9g Protein

8. <u>Tuscan Stewed Beans</u>

Preparation Time: 21 minutes

Cooking Time: 33 minutes

Servings: 1

Ingredients

- 1 dl. extra virgin olive oil

- Salt to taste

- Pepper as needed.

- Cannellini beans

- Sage

- Garlic clove

- Water

Directions

1. Submerge beans for at least 12 hours before cooking.

   Pour the beans in a crockpot with water, a clove of

garlic, sage, and a generous pinch of salt, adjust the flame as low as possible.

2. Once boiling, cover the pot, and continue cooking for at least 3 and a half hours, taking care that the flame remains very low, the beans in the pot must not move around.

3. Once you are done cooking, serve the beans with extra virgin olive oil, salt, and pepper on the table.

Nutrition: 145 Calories 22g fats 15g protein

9. <u>Buckwheat Tabbouleh with Strawberries</u>

Preparation Time: 21 minutes

Cooking Time: 33 minutes

Servings: 1

Ingredients

- Buckwheat (broken)

- Turmeric powder 2 teaspoon

- Avocado 1

- Tomatoes

- Tropia red onions

- Medjool dates (pitted)

- Parsley

- Strawberries

- 2 tablespoons extra virgin olive oil

- Lemon juice 1

- Rocket 1.3 ounce

Direction

1. Heat up the water to cook the buckwheat.

2. When it boils, add turmeric and buckwheat. Be careful not to overcook it. It is good to leave, it "al dente." When cooked, drain the buckwheat and set aside to cool. Take a large bowl to spice the tabbouleh.

3. Cut the tomatoes into cubes and let them drain for a few minutes in a colander to remove the water.

4. On a cutting board, begin to finely chop the red onion, dates, and parsley and combine them with buckwheat.

5. Skin the avocado and cut it into small cubes and add it with the tomatoes to the buckwheat. Cut the strawberries into slices and gently add them to the rest of the ingredients. Add the chopped arugula, oil, and lemon juice. Mix all the ingredients and let the

buckwheat tabbouleh take on extra flavor for an hour

before serving it at the table.

Nutrition: 145 Calories 26g fat 13g protein

10.Scramble Tofu and Mushroom

Preparation Time: 11 minutes

Cooking Time: 28 minutes

Servings: 2

Ingredients

- 7 ounces of extra firm tofu

- 2 teaspoon turmeric powder

- 1 teaspoon black pepper

- ounce of kale, roughly chopped

- 2 teaspoons extra virgin olive oil

- Oz. of red onion

- 1 Thai chili

- 100g mushrooms

- 4 tbsp. parsley

Direction

1. Drain tofu in paper towels.

2. Blend the turmeric with water.

3. Steam the kale for 3 minutes.

4. Cook olive oil at medium heat, fry onion, chili, and mushrooms for 3 minutes

5. Crush the tofu into bite-size pieces and put in the pan, mix the turmeric paste over the tofu. Season with black pepper. Cook at medium heat for 2 minutes

6. Cook kale at medium heat for 4 minutes. Sprinkle parsley and serve.

Nutrition: 122 calories 20g fat 11g protein

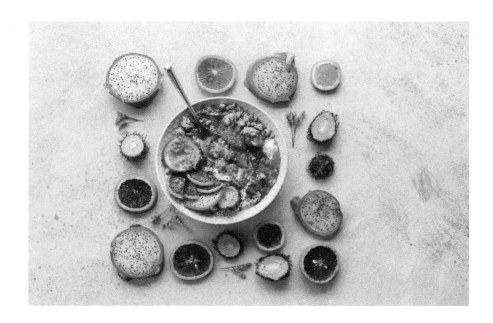

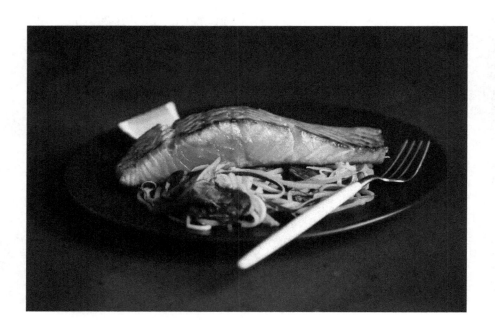

MAIN DISH RECIPES

11. Bacon and Egg Fried Rice

Preparation Time: 18 minutes

Cooking Time: 34 minutes

Servings: 4

Ingredients:

- 350g long-grain rice, well rinsed

- 1 1/2 tablespoon olive oil

- 100g streaky bacon, diced 2 eggs

- Two peppers, finely chopped

- 2 red onions, finely chopped

- 200g carrots, peeled and coarsely grated

- 5cm slice ginger, peeled and grated

- 1 red chili, finely chopped (optional)

- 2 tsp soy sauce

- 2 garlic cloves, crushed

Directions:

1. Cook the rice in a big bowl of warm water for 10 mins until not quite tender. Drain, rinse with warm water and drain. Set aside.

2. Meanwhile, warm 1/2 tablespoon oil in a skillet on a high heat and fry the bacon for 5 - 7 mins until golden and crispy. Remove from the pan using a slotted spoon and place a side. Add 1 tablespoon oil and fry the peppers for 10 mins until lightly bubbling. Add the carrots, onions, ginger, garlic and chili and fry over a moderate - high temperature for 5 mins more.

3. Insert the rice and bacon and simmer for 5 mins, stirring often. Push the rice mix to a single side of this pan and then crack the eggs to the gap. Beat the eggs with a wooden spoon, then stir throughout the rice. Cook for 2 mins, then add the soy sauce and then

remove from heat. Split between 4 shallow bowls to function.

Nutrition: 309 Calories 20g fat 45g Protein

12.Lentil, Kale, and Red Onion Pasta

Preparation Time: 8 minutes

Cooking Time: 35 minutes

Serving: 2

Ingredients

- 2 ½ cups vegetable broth

- ¾ cup dry lentils

- 1 bay leaf

- ¼ cup olive oil

- 1 large red onion, chopped

- 1 teaspoon fresh thyme, chopped

- ½ teaspoon fresh oregano, chopped

- 8 ounces ground turkey, (optional)

- 1 bunch kale

- 1 (12 oz) package buckwheat pasta

- 2 tablespoons nutritional yeast

Directions

1. Rinse the lentils using fine mesh sieve under cold water until the water runs clear

2. Boil vegetable broth, lentils, ½ teaspoon of salt, and bay leaf over high heat. Set heat to medium-low, cover, and cook for 20 minutes. Pour additional broth if needed to keep the lentils moist. Take out the bay leaf once done.

3. As it simmers, cook olive oil in a skillet over medium-high heat. Stir in the onion, thyme, oregano, and season well.

4. Cook for a minute, stirring frequently, then stir ground turkey, if using. Reduce the heat to medium-low, and cook until the onion has softened, about 10 minutes.

5. Meanwhile, bring a large pot of lightly salted water to a boil over high heat. Add the kale and pasta. Cook until the pasta is al dente, about 8 minutes.

6. Remove some of the cooking water and set aside. Drain the pasta, then return to the pot.

7. Stir in the lentils, and onion mixture.

8. Use the reserved cooking liquid to adjust the sauciness of the dish to your liking. Sprinkle with nutritional yeast to serve

Nutrition: 319 Calories 23g fat 42g Protein

13.Pasta with Cheesy Meat Sauce

Preparation Time: 17 minutes

Cooking Time: 26 minutes

Servings: 6

Ingredients:

- ½ box large-shaped pasta

- 1-pound ground beef

- ½ cup onions

- 1 tbsp. onion flakes

- 1½ cups beef stock

- 1 tbsp. Better Than Bouillon® beef

- 1 tablespoon tomato sauce, no salt added

- ¾ cup Monterey or pepper jack cheese, shredded

- 8 ounces cream cheese, softened

- ½ teaspoon Italian seasoning

- ½ teaspoon ground black pepper

- 2 tablespoons French's® Worcestershire sauce, reduced sodium

Direction

1. Cook pasta noodles following the directions on the box.

2. In a sauté pan, fry ground beef, onions and onion flakes until the meat is browned.

3. Strain and add stock, bouillon and tomato sauce.

4. Simmer, stirring occasionally. Put in cooked pasta, turn off heat, and mix softened cream cheese, shredded cheese and seasonings. Stir pasta mixture.

Nutrition: 502 Calories 30g Fat 23g Protein

14.Aromatic Herbed Rice

Preparation Time: 14 minutes

Cooking Time: 18 minutes

Servings: 6

Ingredients:

- 2 tablespoons olive oil

- 3 cups cooked rice (don't overcook)

- 4–5 cloves fresh garlic, sliced thin

- 2 tablespoons fresh cilantro, chopped

- 2 tablespoons fresh oregano, chopped

- 2 tablespoons fresh chives, chopped

- ½ teaspoon red pepper flakes

- 1 teaspoon red wine vinegar

Directions:

1. In a large sauté pan, heat olive oil on medium-high heat and lightly sauté garlic. Add rice, herbs and red

pepper flakes and continue to cook for 2–4 minutes or until well-mixed.

2. Turn off heat, add vinegar, mix well and serve.

Nutrition: 134 Calories 5g Fat 2g Protein

15.Herb-Crusted Roast Leg of Lamb

Preparation Time: 17 minutes

Cooking Time: 38 minutes

Servings: 12

Ingredients:

- 1 4-pound leg of lamb

- 3 tablespoons lemon juice

- 1 tablespoon curry powder

- 2 cloves garlic, minced

- ½ teaspoon ground black pepper

- 1 cup onions, sliced

- ½ cup dry vermouth

Direction:

1. Prep oven to 400° F.

2. Situate leg of lamb on a roasting pan. Drizzle 1 tsp. of

   lemon juice.

3. Blend 2 teaspoons of lemon juice and the rest of the spices. Brush paste onto the lamb.

4. Roast lamb at 400° F for 30 minutes.

5. Strain off fat and stir vermouth and onions.

6. Set heat to 325° F and cook for 2 hours. Baste leg of lamb frequently. Pull out from oven and rest 3 minutes before serving.

Nutrition: 292 Calories 20g Fat 24g Protein

16.Baked Potatoes with Spicy Chickpea

Preparation: 18 minutes Cooking: 9 minutes Servings: 5

Ingredients:

- 4-6 baking potatoes, pricked all over

- Two tablespoons olive oil

- Two red onions, finely chopped

- Four cloves garlic, grated or crushed

- 2cm ginger, grated

- Two tablespoons turmeric

- ½ -2 teaspoons of chili flakes (depending on how hot you like things)

- Two tablespoons cumin seeds

- Splash of water

- Two into 400g tins chopped tomatoes

- Two tablespoons unsweetened cocoa powder (or cacao)

- Two into 400g tins chickpeas (or kidney beans if you prefer) including the chickpea water

- Two yellow peppers (or whatever color you prefer!), chopped into bite size pieces

- Salt and pepper to taste (optional)

- Side salad (optional)

Directions:

1. Preheat the oven to 200C so you can make all the ingredients you need.

2. Put your baking potatoes in the oven when the oven is hot enough, and cook them for an hour or till they are cooked as you want them.

3. Put the olive oil and chopped red onion in a big broad saucepan once the potatoes are in the oven and cook gently with the lid until the onions are soft but not brown for 5 minutes.

4. Remove the lid and add the garlic, cumin, ginger and chili. Cook on low heat for another minute, and then you add the turmeric and a tiny drizzle of water and cook for 3 minutes, keeping in minute not to let the saucepan get too dry.

5. Add cocoa (or cacao) powder, chickpeas (including chickpea water) and yellow pepper in the tomatoes. Boil it and simmer for 45 minutes at low heat until the sauce is thick and greasy (but don't let it burn!). Stew will be handled roughly at the same time as the potatoes.

6. At last, mix in the two tablespoons of parsley and some salt and pepper, if desired, and serve the stew over the baked potatoes, maybe with a small side salad.

Nutrition: 243 Calories 24g Fat 16g Protein

17.Buckwheat with Red Onion Dal

Preparation Time: 8 minutes

Cooking Time: 0 minutes

Servings: 4

Ingredients:

- One tablespoon olive oil

- One small red onion, sliced

- Three garlic cloves, grated or crushed

- One bird eye chili deseeded and finely chopped (more if you like things hot!)

- 2 cm ginger, grated

- Two teaspoons turmeric

- Two teaspoons graham masala

- 160g red lentils

- 200ml water

- 400ml coconut milk

- 160g buckwheat (or brown rice)

- 100g kale

Directions:

1. In a big, deep saucepan, put the olive oil and add the sliced onion. Cook at low pressure, with the lid on until softened for 5 minutes.

2. Add the garlic, chili and ginger and cook for 1 minute.

3. Add the turmeric, graham masala, sprinkle with water and cook for 1 minute.

4. Add the red lentils, coconut milk and 200 ml of water (fill the coconut milk with water and drop it into the casserole).

5. Thoroughly mix everything and cook over a gentle heat for 20 minutes with the lid on. If the dhal starts sticking, stir periodically and add a little more water.

6. After 20 minutes, add the Kale, whisk thoroughly and remove the lid and cook for another 5 minutes (1-2 minutes if spinach is used instead!)

7. Place the buckwheat in a medium saucepan about 15 minutes before the curry is ready, and put plenty of boiling water. Bring the water again to the boil and cook for 10 minutes

Nutrition: 234 Calories 19g fat 9g protein

SIDES RECIPES

18. Quinoa and Peas

Preparation Time: 12 minutes

Cooking Time: 34 minutes

Servings: 4

Ingredients:

- 1 yellow onion, chopped

- 1 tomato, cubed

- 1 cup quinoa

- 3 cups vegetable stock

- 1 tablespoon olive oil   1 cup peas

- 1 tablespoon cilantro, chopped

- A pinch of salt and black pepper

Directions:

1. Heat up a pot with the oil over medium heat, add the onion, stir and sauté for 5 minutes.

2. Add the quinoa, the stock and the other ingredients, toss, bring to a simmer and cook over medium heat for 25 minutes.

3. Divide everything between plates and serve as a side dish.

Nutrition: 202 calories 3g fat 6g protein

19.Lemon Splash Tofu

Preparation Time: 9 minutes

Cooking Time: 13 minutes

Serving: 3

Ingredients:

- 250 grams firm tofu – extra firm

- ½ teaspoon lemon zest – freshly grated

- ¼ lemon – peeled, fresh

- 1/8 cup sundried tomatoes

- 1 garlic clove

- ½ teaspoon ground fennel seeds

- 1 tablespoon extra-virgin olive oil

Direction:

1. Prepare the oven to 400 degrees F. Combine olive oil, tomatoes, fennel, crushed garlic, and lemon zest to

make a marinade for the tofu. Lightly oil a baking dish then cut the tofu into four equal pieces.

2. Coat the top of the pieces with some of the marinade. Arrange the pieces in the baking dish. Bake for 13 minutes. Serve with the rest of the marinade and enjoy your dish.

Nutrition: 254 Calories 20g Fat 14g Protein

20. <u>**Veggie Stuffed Peppers**</u>

Preparation Time: 14 minutes

Cooking Time: 36 minutes

Serving: 6

Ingredients:

- 1 green pepper

- ¾ cup brown rice - cooked

- 2 tablespoons red onion – diced

- 2 tablespoons celery – diced

- ¼ cup tomato puree

- ½ bird's eye chili – finely sliced

- ½ teaspoon oregano - dry

- ½ teaspoon basil – dry

- ½ teaspoon thyme – ground

- 2 slices Mozzarella cheese

- 2 tablespoons olive oil

Directions:

1. Preheat skillet with a tablespoon of olive oil on medium heat. Add onions and celery and diced green pepper to the skillet. Sauté for one to two minutes.

2. Add tomato puree then cook for five minutes while simmering. Add the herbs and spices and stir in to combine. Add the brown rice and stir in to combine all the ingredients.

3. Take the whole pepper – top off and deseeded - and cut it in half across the length. Stuff each half with rice mixture. Situate one slice of cheese on each half then place in a lightly greased up baking dish. Bake over 350 degrees F for 23 minutes. Serve and enjoy!

Nutrition: 405 Calories 15g Fat 18g Protein

21.Veggie Jambalaya

Preparation Time: 12 minutes

Cooking Time: 29 minutes

Serving: 3

Ingredients:

- ¼ cup dark red beans – canned

- ¼ cup red onion – chop

- ¼ cup red bell pepper – chopped

- ¼ cup yellow pepper – chopped

- ¾ cups brown rice - cooked

- 1 garlic clove – minced

- 50 grams tomato paste – canned

- 25 grams silk five-grain tempeh

- ½ cup vegetable broth

- 1 bird's eye chili pepper

- 1 tablespoon extra-virgin olive oil

- Salt to taste

Directions:

1. Prep skillet on medium-high heat and add the oil. Add garlic and onion and sauté for a minute or two.

2. Reduce the heat to medium. Add sliced tempeh and peppers and cook until the veggies are softened to your preference. Add the spices and salt, broth, and tomato paste. Stir in to combine then bring the mixture to a simmer.

3. Once the jambalaya starts to simmer, add cooked brown rice and stir to combine. Serve while hot and enjoy your lunch.

Nutrition: 509 Calories 16g Fat 15g Protein

SEAFOOD RECIPES

22.   <u>Smoked Salmon Pasta</u>

Preparation Time: 14 minutes

Cooking Time: 23 minutes

Serving: 4

Ingredients

- Extra virgin olive oil 2 tablespoons

- Red onion, finely sliced 1

- Garlic cloves, finely sliced 2

- Thai chilies, finely sliced 2

- Cherry tomatoes, cut in half 1 cup

- White wine 1/2 cup

- Buckwheat pasta 9 to 11 ounces

- Smoked salmon 9 ounces

- Capers   2 tablespoons

- Juice of lemon   ½

- Arugula 2 ounces

- Parsley, chopped 1/4 cup

Direction

1. In a broiler pan start cooking one teaspoon of the oil over moderate flame. Stir in the onion, garlic, chili, and fry till smooth but not dark brown.

2. Start adding the tomatoes and permit to bake for one or two minutes. To minimize by half, append the white wine and bubble.

3. Bake the pasta in hot water with one tablespoon of oil for eight to ten minutes based on whether you like it to serve, then rinse.

4. Split the salmon into pieces and apply the capers, lemon juice, arugula, parsley, and the tomato into saucepan. Insert the sauce, blend together, and eat straight away. Sprinkle some oil over top.

Nutrition: 334 Calories 21g Fat 13g Protein

23. Vietnamese Turmeric Fish with Herbs & Mango Sauce

Preparation: 23 minutesCooking: 34 minutes Serving:4

Ingredients

- Fresh cod fish 1 ¼ lbs.

- Coconut oil in pan and fry the fish 2 tablespoons

- Sea salt to taste

Fish marinade

- Turmeric powder 1 tablespoon

- Sea salt 1 teaspoon

- Chinese cooking wine 1 tablespoon

- Minced ginger 2 teaspoons

- Olive oil 2 tablespoons

Infused Scallion and Dill Oil

- Scallions 2 cups Fresh dill 2 cups

- Sea salt to taste Mango dipping sauce

- Medium sized ripe mango 1

- Rice vinegar 2 tablespoons

- Juice of lime ½

- Garlic clove 1

- Dry red chili pepper 1 teaspoon

Direction

1. Marinate the fish for one hour or as long as it is overnight.

2. Add all ingredients in a mixing bowl under "Mango Dipping Sauce," and combine until quality is obtained.

For the Fish:

3. Cook 2 tablespoons of coconut oil at high temperature in a big, nonstick skillet. Add the pre-marinated fish if hot

4. A loud sizzle should be heard, upon which you can reduce the heat to moderate heat.

5. Do not turn or relocate the fish till after, about 5 minutes. Top with a tablespoon of sea salt.

6. When the fish is in golden brown, move the fish gently on the other side on cook. Transmit onto a large plate once it's accomplished.

For Scallion and Dill Infused Oil:

7. Just use rest of the oil over medium to high heat in the frying pan, stir in 2 cups of scallions and 2 cups of dill. Remove from the heat once the scallions and dill are introduced. Start giving them a delicate flip, about fifteen seconds, till the scallions and dill simmered. Season with a sprinkle of salt at sea.

8. Plop the scallion, dill and infused oil over the fish and represent fresh cilantro, lime, and nuts with mango sauce.

Nutrition: 471 Calories 31g Fat 21g Protein

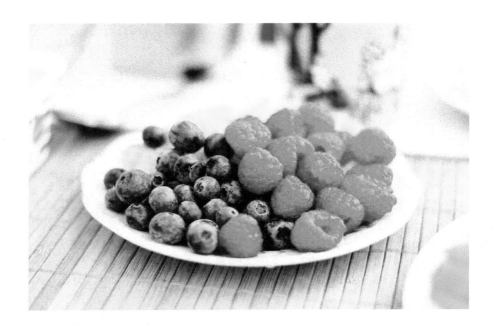

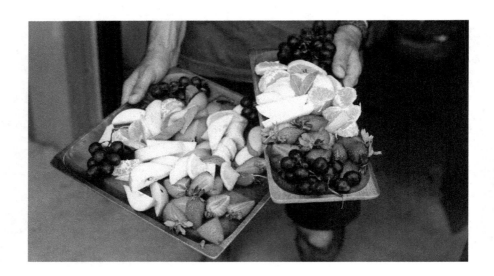

VEGETABLE RECIPES

24.   Cucumber Bites with Salmon and Avocado

Preparation Time: 22 minutes

Cooking Time: 13 minutes

Servings: 2

Ingredients:

- Black pepper for garnish

- 6 oz. Smoked salmon

- ½ tbsp. Lime juice

- ¼ c. Red onion, chopped

- 1 Cucumber

- 1 Avocado peel and remove the pit

Directions:

1. Peel the cucumber if and then slice it into slices that are about one-fourth inch thick, and then put the slices on a plate for serving.

2. Cream together the lime juice and avocado until they are creamy and smooth. Put a teaspoon of the mashed avocado on each slice of cucumber, and then top the avocado with a slice of the smoked salmon.

3. Use the onions and black pepper to garnish as you like.

Nutrition: 278 Calories 27g Protein 19g Fat

25.   **Butter Bean and Vegetable Korma**

Preparation Time: 9 minutes

Cooking Time: 34 minutes

Serving: 4

Ingredients

- three normal-size cloves of garlic

- one onion

- one fresh chili

- ½ piece of fresh ginger, thumb size

- 750g sweet potatoes

- one medium tomato

- 250g frozen peas

- 100g green sugar snaps/beans

- 2 tbsp. oil

- 400g large leek

- 400ml water

- one tin (400ml) coconut milk

- 3 tbsp. soy sauce/tamari

- 1 tbsp. honey

- 2 tsp. ground cumin

- Juice of a lemon

- 2 tsp. ground coriander

- 1 tsp. ground turmeric

- 2 tsp. salt

- 4 tsp. medium curry powder

- ½ tsp. freshly ground black pepper

- Bunch of fresh coriander

- one tin (400g) butterbeans

Direction

1. Pour two tablespoons of oil into a huge saucepan. Chop the tomato, red onion and put them into the pan

2. Add the grated ginger, chili chopped garlic into the pan and have it cooked for about five minutes.

3. Prepare the leeks and sweet potato. Do not forget to include the leafy bits

4. Add the ground cumin, curry powder, turmeric, ground coriander, and black pepper to the pan.

5. Next, add 400 ml of water, one tin of coconut milk, two teaspoons of salt, the juice of 1 lemon, 1tablespoons of liquid sweetener, and three tablespoons of tamari (or soy sauce)

6. Add the leeks, sweet potato, and beans and have the mixture stewed until the sweet potatoes are cooked or for about 20 minutes.

7. Save a few peas for the purpose of garnishing and the rest of it inside. Also, add sugar snap peas. Serve!

Nutrition: 417 calories 19g fats 8g protein

26.   Courgette Tortilla

Preparation Time: 8 minutes Cooking Time: 21 minutes

Serving: 2

Ingredients

- 1 tbsp. olive oil

- one large coarsely grated courgette

- 1 tsp. harissa

- four large eggs

- 3 tbsps. reduced-fat hummus

- one large red pepper, torn into strips

- three pitted queen olives, quartered

- Handful coriander

Direction

1. Cook oil in a 20cm non-stick frying pan. Put the courgette and let it cook for some minute while stirring it periodically until it softens.

2. Beat the eggs with the harissa and pour them into the pan.

3. Proceed to cook gently. Stir to let the egg that is uncooked flow onto the base of the pan.

4. When more than half has been cooked, do not touch it for about two minutes. Place a plate, then take back to the pan, facing the uncooked part down, to have the cooking completed.

5. Tip on top of a board and spread using the hummus to serve.

6. Scatter with the coriander, olives, and pepper.

7. Cut into quarters and eat cold or warm.

Nutrition: 317 calories 21g fat 13g protein

27. **Almond Butter and Alfalfa Wraps**

Preparation Time: 7 minutes

Cooking Time: 0 minutes

Servings: 1

Ingredients

- Juice of 1 lemon

- 4 tbsp. of almond nut butter

- three finely sliced radishes

- 2-3 carrots grated

- 1 cup of alfalfa sprouts

- Nori sheets or lettuce leaves

- Pepper and salt

Direction

1. Combine the almond butter with a sufficient amount of water and an ample amount of lemon juice so you will have a paste with your desired level of thickness.

2. Next, have the alfalfa sprouts and grated carrot mixed inside a bowl. Sprinkle with the remaining lemon juice that was set aside. Proceed to the season with pepper and salt to taste.

3. Using the almond butter, smear the nori sheets or lettuce leaves, depending on the one you are using. Top the resulting mixture with the alfalfa sprout mixture and carrot. Roll it up and serve. Enjoy!

Nutrition: 409 calories 17g fat 6g protein

28. <u>Buckwheat Bean and Tomato Risotto</u>

Preparation: 11 minutes Cooking: 23 minutesServings: 4

Ingredients

- 2 tbsp. of butter or olive oil

- two cloves of chopped garlic

- eight ounces/225g buckwheat

- 400ml of vegetable stock or hot water

- eight ounces/225g broad beans

- ½ cup of sun-dried tomatoes inside an oil

- Juice of half a lemon

- 2 tbsp. of chopped coriander or basil

- two ounces/50g of toasted almonds Pepper and salt

Direction

1. Heat the butter or olive oil inside a frying pan. Include the garlic and allow it to cook for a period of one minute.

2. Next, place the buckwheat into the pan and have it stirred thoroughly. This is to allow the buckwheat to be coated in the oil.

3. After that, add the stock or hot water. Then close the frying pan and let it simmer for 10 minutes.

4. When you are done simmering, stir the broad beans in. Then proceed to cook until the beans are just tender, which should be for a few minutes.

5. After that, add the fresh herbs, lemon juice, sun-dried tomatoes, and almonds. Season with pepper and salt to taste. Serve and enjoy your meal!

Nutrition: 358 calories 21g fat 14g protein

29.   <u>Vegetable Curry with Tofu</u>

Preparation Time: 14 minutes

Cooking Time: 20 minutes

Serving: 3

Ingredients

- ½ tbsp. rapeseed oil

- One large onion, chopped

- three cloves garlic, peeled and grated

- One large thumb (7cm) fresh ginger, peeled and grated

- One red chili, deseeded and thinly sliced

- ¼ tsp ground turmeric

- ¼ tsp cayenne pepper

- ½ tsp paprika

- ¼ tsp ground cumin

- ½ tsp salt

- 150g dried red lentils

- ½ -liter boiling water

- 30g frozen soya edamame beans

- 100g firm tofu, chopped into cubes

- a tomato, roughly chopped

- Juice of 1 lime

- 100g kale leaves stalk removed and torn

Direction

1. Put the oil over low-medium heat in a heavy-bottom pan. Add the turmeric, cayenne, cumin, paprika, and oil. Remove and mix again before adding the red lentils.

2. Pour in the boiling water and cook for 10 minutes until the curry has a thick' porridge' consistency, then reduce the heat and cook for another 20-30 minutes.

3. Add soya beans, tofu, and tomatoes and continue to
    cook for another 5 minutes. Add the juice of lime and
    kale leaves and cook until the kale is tender.

Nutrition 342 Calories 5g Fat 28g Protein

SOUP AND STEW RECIPES

30. Curry and Rice Stew

Preparation Time: 12 minutes

Cooking Time: 17 minutes

Serving: 4

Ingredients:

- 2 teaspoons of rapeseed oil

- 225 g paneer, cut into cubes

- Salt and freshly ground black pepper

- 1 red onion, sliced

- 1 thumb (5 cm) fresh ginger, peeled and grated

- 2 cloves of garlic, peeled and grated

- 2 fingers of chili peppers, heads removed and finely chopped

- ½ teaspoon aniseed

- 250 g cooked brown rice

- 250 g ready-to-eat or cooked Puy lentils

- 100 g frozen soy / edamame beans

- ½ teaspoon salt

- ½ teaspoon ground turmeric

- ½ teaspoon ground cumin

- ½ teaspoon ground coriander

- 1 teaspoon mild chili powder

- 2 tomatoes, chopped

- 50g baby spinach leaves

- Large handful (20g) parsley, chopped

Direction:

1. Cook oil in a large pan over high heat and add the paneer. Season generously with salt and pepper.

2. Cook the paneer, stirring frequently, until golden brown all over. Pull out and set aside.

3. Add the onion and reduce the heat in the pan to low. Before adding the ginger, garlic, chili peppers and anise, cook for 2 minutes and cook slowly for another 5 minutes.

4. Put the rice and lentils in a large bowl and mix gently, breaking up any lumps and separating the grains.

5. If the soybeans are frozen or need to be cooked, cook them according to the directions in the package. Add the salt, ground spices and chili powder to the pan and stir. Add the rice and lentil mixture, soybeans and tomatoes to the pan.

6. Stir very well and cook hot. Finally add the spinach and parsley and return the paneer to the pan.

7. Stir to combine and serve immediately. After cooling down completely, all spare servings can be chilled and served cold the next day.

Nutrition 19g Fat 24g Protein 347 Calories

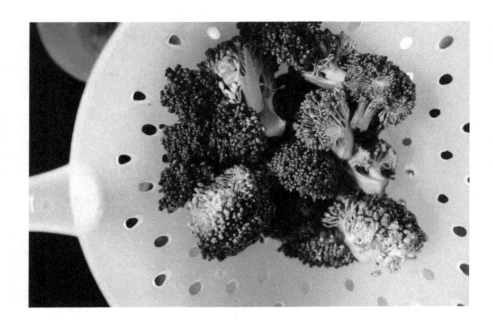

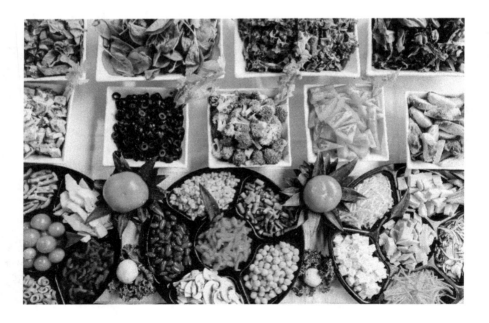

VEGETARIAN RECIPES

31.Mediterranean Sirtfood Quinoa

Preparation Time: 16 minutes

Cooking Time: 29 minutes

Serving: 5

Ingredients:

- Quinoa, 2 cups

- Extra virgin olive oil, 1 tbsp

- Finely chopped garlic cloves, 1 tbsp

- Fresh ginger, chopped, 1 tsp

- 1 sliced bird's eye chili

- 1 sliced red bell pepper

- Ground turmeric, ½ tsp

- Ground cumin, 1 tsp

- A pinch of salt

- A pinch of pepper

- Chopped kale, 1 cup

- Lemon juice, 2 tbsp

Direction:

1. Start off by cooking the quinoa. Pour into a pot, cover with two parts water, and bring to a boil. Let it boil for up to thirty minutes.

2. During the last five minutes, pan-fry the vegetables except kale in olive oil for up to five minutes. Once the vegetables have softened, add cumin, paprika, turmeric, salt, and pepper.

3. Stir through and insert quinoa. Stir again, add vegetable stock, and pan-fry until the excess liquid vapors out. Serve and enjoy!

Nutrition: 487 calories 31g fats 24g protein

SALAD RECIPES

32.   Carrot, Buckwheat, Tomato & Arugula

Salad in a Jar

Preparation Time: 16 minutes

Cooking Time: 0 minute

Serving: 2

Ingredients

- 1/2 cup sunflower seeds

- 1/2 cup carrots

- 1/2 cup of shredded cabbage

- 1/2 cup of tomatoes

- 1 cup cooked buckwheat mixed with 1 tbsp. chia seeds

- 1 cup arugula

Dressing:

- 1 tbsp. olive oil

- 1 tbsp. fresh lemon juice and pinch of sea salt

Direction:

1. Put ingredients in this order: dressing, sunflower seeds, carrots, cabbage, tomatoes, buckwheat and arugula.

Nutrition: 201 Calories 3g Fat 6g Protein

33.   Chickpeas, Onion, Tomato & Parsley Salad in a Jar

Preparation Time: 9 minutes Cooking Time: 0 minute

Serving: 2

Ingredients

- 1 cup cooked chickpeas

- 1/2 cup chopped tomatoes

- 1/2 of a small onion, chopped

- 1 tbsp. chia seeds 1 Tbsp. chopped parsley

Dressing:

- 1 tbsp. olive oil and 1 tbsp. of Chlorella.

- 1 tbsp. fresh lemon juice and pinch of sea salt

Direction:

1. Put ingredients in this order: dressing, tomatoes, chickpeas, onions and parsley.

Nutrition: 253 Calories 8g Fat 5g Protein

34. <u>Arugula, Carrot, Corn & Spinach Salad in a Jar</u>

Preparation Time: 11 minutes Cooking Time: 0 minute

Serving: 2

Ingredients

- 1 cup corn

- 1 cup tomatoes

- 1/2 cup of julienned carrot

- 1/2 cup arugula

Dressing:

- 1 tbsp. olive oil 2 Tbsp. Greek Yogurt

- 1 tbsp. fresh lemon juice and pinch of sea salt

Direction:

1. Put ingredients in this order: dressing, tomatoes, corn, carrots, and arugula.

Nutrition: 247 Calories 8.3g Fat 4g Protein

35.   **Greek Stuffed Portobello Mushrooms**

Preparation Time: 1 hour Cooking Time: 42 minutes

Servings: 4

Ingredients:

- 3 tablespoons extra-virgin olive oil, divided

- ½ teaspoon ground pepper, divided

- 1 cup chopped spinach

- ½ cup quartered cherry tomatoes

- 1 clove garlic, minced

- ¼ teaspoon salt

- 2 tablespoons pitted and sliced Kalamata olives

- 4 Portobello mushrooms

- 1/3 cup crumbled feta cheese

- 1 tablespoon chopped fresh oregano

Directions:

1. Firstly, Preheat oven to 400 degrees F.

2. Mix 2 tablespoons oil, garlic, 1/4 teaspoon pepper and salt in a small bowl. Using a silicone brush, coat mushrooms all over with the oil mixture. Place on a large rimmed baking sheet and bake until the mushrooms are mostly soft, 8 to 10 minutes.

3. In the meantime, combine spinach, tomatoes, feta, olives, oregano and the remaining 1 tablespoon oil in a medium bowl. Once the mushrooms have softened, remove from the oven and fill with the spinach mixture. Bake until the tomatoes have wilted, about 10 minutes.

Nutrition: 345 Calories 54g Fat 6g Protein

36.   <u>Turmeric Sautéed Greens</u>

Preparation Time: 3 minutes

Cooking Time: 0 minutes

Servings: 3

Ingredients:

- 1 tablespoon olive oil

- 1 2-inch piece fresh turmeric

- 1/4 teaspoon kosher salt

- 3 garlic cloves, minced

- 2 tablespoons water

- 2 bunches kale, spinach, or Swiss chard, thinly sliced

Directions:

1. Firstly, heat oil in a large sauce pan by using medium heat.

2. Now, add garlic and turmeric and sauté for 30 seconds.

3. Further, add kale and salt and sauté for 1 minute.

4. At the last add water to the pan and cook stirring until the greens are just wilted and serve.

Nutrition: 87 Calories 56g Protein 28g fat

37.   Sautéed Collard Greens

Preparation Time: 21 minutes

Cooking Time: 17 minutes

Servings: 4

Ingredients:

- 1 slice thick-cut bacon, diced

- 1 bunch collard greens

- 2 garlic cloves, minced

- 1/2 teaspoon kosher salt

Directions:

1. Firstly, Put the bacon in a sauté pan over medium-low heat and cook for 5 minutes to render as much fat as possible.

2. While the bacon is cooking, remove the stems from the collard greens, and thinly slice the leaves across.

3. Now, add the garlic to the pan and cook for 1 minute. Add the greens and salt, stir well to coat the greens

with the bacon fat, reduce heat to low, and cook for 5 minutes, until wilted, stirring occasionally. If you like them softer, cook for 10 minutes.

Nutrition: 87 Calories 10g Fat 56g Protein

DESSERT RECIPES

38.   Brazil Nut Brittle

Preparation Time: 11 minutes

Cooking Time: 3 minutes

Serving: 6

Ingredients

- 150g (5oz) Brazil nuts, chopped

- 150g (5oz) dark chocolate (min 70% cocoa)

Direction:

1. Double-boil the chocolate in a bowl then over a saucepan of lightly simmering water and let it melt. In the meantime, place half of the chopped Brazil nuts in the bottom of a small dish or small loaf tin. When the chocolate has melted and is smooth, pour half of it over the chopped nuts.

2. Add in the remaining chopped nuts and pour over the remaining melted chocolate. Chill in the fridge until it hardens. Break the brittle into chunks and serve.

Nutrition: 322 Calories 18g Protein 15g Fat

39. **Strawberry Buckwheat Pancakes**

Preparation Time: 7 minutes

Cooking Time: 42 minutes

Servings: 2

Ingredients:

- 100g 3½oz strawberries, chopped

- 100g 3½ oz. buckwheat flour

- 1 egg

- 250mls 8fl oz. milk

- 1 teaspoon olive oil

- 1 teaspoon olive oil for frying

- Freshly squeezed juice of 1 orange

Directions:

1. Pour the milk. Mix in the egg and olive oil. Sift in the flour to the liquid mixture. Heat a little oil in a pan

and pour in a quarter of the mixture or to the size you prefer.

2. Sprinkle in a quarter of the strawberries into the batter. Cook for around 2 minutes on each side. Serve hot with a drizzle of orange juice.

Nutrition: 175 Calories 35g Fat 21g Protein

40.   <u>Strawberry & Nut Granola</u>

Preparation Time: 7 minutes

Cooking Time: 51 minutes

Servings: 2

Ingredients:

- 200g 7oz oats

- 250g 9oz buckwheat flakes

- 100g 3½ oz. walnuts, chopped

- 100g 3½ oz. almonds, chopped

- 100g 3½ oz. dried strawberries

- 1½ teaspoons ground ginger

- 1½ teaspoons ground cinnamon

- 120mls 4fl oz. olive oil 2 tablespoon honey

Directions:

1. Combine the oats, buckwheat flakes, nuts, ginger and cinnamon.

2. In a saucepan, warm the oil and honey. Stir until the honey has melted.

3. Pour the warm oil into the dry ingredients and mix well.

4. Fill mixture out on a big baking tray and bake at 300F until the granola is golden.

5. Allow it to cool. Add in the dried berries. Store in an airtight container until ready to use.

Nutrition: 360 Calories 28g Fat 19g Protein

CONCLUSION

Thanks for making it to the end of sirtfood diet cookbook. Sirtfood diet plan is a great plan that like all plans need to be implemented with a great deal of effort, discipline and determination. Sirtfood diet can help you lose weight if you fully implement it into your life and make it a habit.

As stated above this diet is not supposed to be a short-term plan but a long-term lifestyle goal. You cannot implement this diet and then revert to your normal eating habits. You need to adopt lifestyle changes. If you wish to lose weight and stay fit, then you need to do something about it.

It is suggested to eat sirtfood diet recipes every day. The future benefits of sirtfood diet will overcome any initial discomfort you might feel during the beginning phases of the diet. If you wish to make this diet successful, then you need to believe in it.

I hope you have enjoyed reading Sirtfood Diet Plan.

Good luck on your sirtfood journey!

CPSIA information can be obtained
at www.ICGtesting.com
Printed in the USA
BVHW090808030621
608729BV00002B/372